Holy sh*t

I need a NEW ME!

◇

A 90 DAY FOOD & EXERCISE
TRACKER FOR PEOPLE
in need of change

**TANGO
CHARLIE**

Holy sh*t, I need a new me

We've all been there. Squished in some horrendous changing room trying to avoid eye contact with the mirror as you squeeze yourself into a pair of jeans or wrestle your boobs into a new top, only to get depressed when nothing fits, leave the store in a grump and head to the cafe to 'cheer yourself up' with a slice of cake.

But hang on a minute Droopy Doris, you're reading this page which means something in your head has gone **"Hang on, I'm a bit sick of this sh*t... I need to do something about it!"**

Which means you've bought this book (clearly you're a genius) and you're committed to changing your habits for the next 90 days, tracking everything you eat, and writing down any exercise you do (or pretend to do). You know you need to start **taking control somewhere**, and this journal is the bloody right place to start.

So, read over the next few pages for tips and suggestions, write down body measurements (preferably yours!) so you can be that impressive 'transformation winner' you always see on Instagram, and
let's get this sh*t started!

(Feel free to roar like a lion now)

Sort your sh*t out

Below are some things you can start doing RIGHT NOW which will help you on this 90 day journey. Some tips will help your waistline; others will help your mind. ALL will help you get started.

01 **If you bite it - write it.** When food passes your lips, write it down! Even if it will make you feel guilty afterwards. By having it listed in this book, you'll be more likely to stick to healthy foods.

02 **Avoid processed foods.** Its all junk and you deserve better than that. The sneaky manufacturers put loads of sugar and sh*t in processed stuff.

03 **Drink loads of water.** Or a green tea. But NOT fizzy soda or sweetened juices. Red wine is reportedly "good for your heart" but pretty sure you can go without it for 90 days. Pfft... who am I kidding? Just remember to WRITE IT DOWN!

04 Do not judge yourself. **"I f*cken rock"** is your new mantra.

05 Eat more natural food like fruit and veg. **The greener, the better.** Experiment with things you've never tried. You got in this state by bad habits, so make some new healthy ones!

06 If you're bored, **get active.** Preferably a walk outside (away from the pantry). Ride a bike, meet a friend for a 'walk and talk', do something that will keep you from being bored. Boredom is NOT your friend.

07 **Use the stairs.** Try and beat the lazy sods on the escalator to the top. Wear your 'smug' face when doing so.

08 **S-t-r-e-t-c-h.** Find a quiet spot each day to stretch your body and increase flexibility. Touch your toes... or your knees, or try a gentle YouTube yoga session ('Yoga with Adriene' is my fav).

09 **Go outside more.** Run around the neighborhood like your granny used to tell you. Go on... off you trot.

10 **Go to bed earlier.** It's like a reverse 'sleeping in' and a real treat!

11 **Dance.** Put on loud music and have a disco at home. Repeat your new mantra from #04 when you're dancing.

12 **Wear clothes that make you happy -** unless Crocs make you happy. Then dump that sh*t. No one needs to see those.

13 **Throw away** things you do not need. (Like those Crocs if you have them). Decluttering can be therapeutic.

14 **Meditate.** This doesn't mean spending hours being zen in odd positions. It can mean to pause a few times a day and do some deep breathing. It's life-changing.

15 **Remember.** Remember why you started this. Remember that all your efforts over the next 90 days will be worth it. Remember it won't kill you if you sweat a little. Remember you're in charge.

Now, let's do this!

Your starting point

DAY 01

Body measurements. They're fun. Not. But by keeping track of your 'New Me' progress, they can be incredibly valuable, and a great motivator to keep going. Use whatever unit you wish to measure your body... remember to be consistent each time you measure and record the numbers.

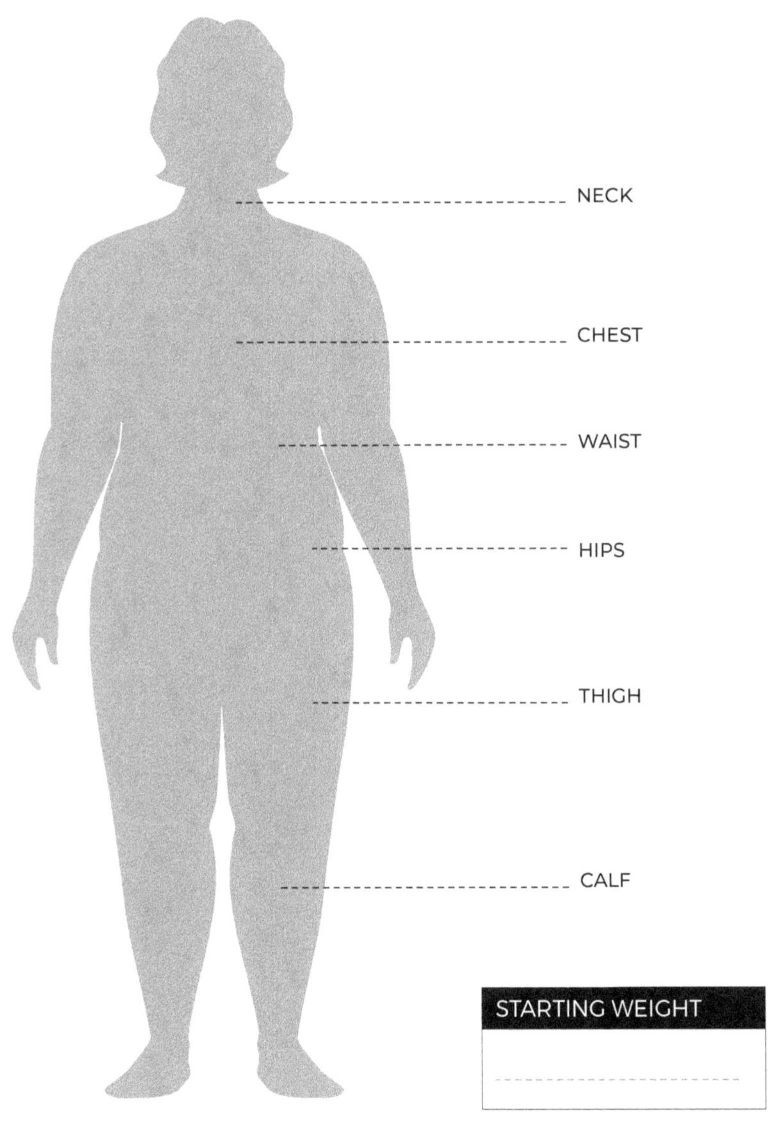

STARTING WEIGHT

Day **01**

BREAKFAST

LUNCH

DINNER

SNACKS

EXERCISE / ACTIVITY

WATER

I SLEPT FOR

HOURS

CHALLENGES I FACED TODAY:

SOMETHING TO MAKE TOMORROW BETTER:

Day 02

BREAKFAST   LUNCH   DINNER

SNACKS

EXERCISE / ACTIVITY

WATER

I SLEPT FOR

HOURS

CHALLENGES I FACED TODAY:

SOMETHING TO MAKE TOMORROW BETTER:

Day **03**

BREAKFAST	LUNCH	DINNER

SNACKS

EXERCISE / ACTIVITY

WATER

I SLEPT FOR

HOURS

CHALLENGES I FACED TODAY:

SOMETHING TO MAKE TOMORROW BETTER:

Day 04

BREAKFAST

LUNCH

DINNER

SNACKS

EXERCISE / ACTIVITY

WATER

I SLEPT FOR

HOURS

CHALLENGES I FACED TODAY:

SOMETHING TO MAKE TOMORROW BETTER:

Day **05**

BREAKFAST   LUNCH   DINNER

SNACKS

EXERCISE / ACTIVITY

WATER

I SLEPT FOR

HOURS

CHALLENGES I FACED TODAY:

SOMETHING TO MAKE TOMORROW BETTER:

Day **06**

BREAKFAST   LUNCH   DINNER

SNACKS

EXERCISE / ACTIVITY

WATER

I SLEPT FOR

HOURS

CHALLENGES I FACED TODAY:

SOMETHING TO MAKE TOMORROW BETTER:

Day 07

BREAKFAST   LUNCH   DINNER

SNACKS

EXERCISE / ACTIVITY

WATER

I SLEPT FOR

HOURS

CHALLENGES I FACED TODAY:

SOMETHING TO MAKE TOMORROW BETTER:

Day **08**

BREAKFAST

LUNCH

DINNER

SNACKS

EXERCISE / ACTIVITY

WATER

I SLEPT FOR

HOURS

CHALLENGES I FACED TODAY:

SOMETHING TO MAKE TOMORROW BETTER:

Day 09

BREAKFAST   LUNCH   DINNER

SNACKS

EXERCISE / ACTIVITY

WATER

I SLEPT FOR

HOURS

CHALLENGES I FACED TODAY:

SOMETHING TO MAKE TOMORROW BETTER:

Day **10**

BREAKFAST

LUNCH

DINNER

SNACKS

EXERCISE / ACTIVITY

WATER

I SLEPT FOR

HOURS

CHALLENGES I FACED TODAY:

SOMETHING TO MAKE TOMORROW BETTER:

Day **11**

BREAKFAST   LUNCH   DINNER

SNACKS

EXERCISE / ACTIVITY

WATER

I SLEPT FOR

HOURS

CHALLENGES I FACED TODAY:

SOMETHING TO MAKE TOMORROW BETTER:

Day **12**

BREAKFAST   LUNCH   DINNER

SNACKS

EXERCISE / ACTIVITY

WATER

I SLEPT FOR

HOURS

CHALLENGES I FACED TODAY:

SOMETHING TO MAKE TOMORROW BETTER:

Day **13**

BREAKFAST   LUNCH   DINNER

SNACKS

EXERCISE / ACTIVITY

WATER

I SLEPT FOR

HOURS

CHALLENGES I FACED TODAY:

SOMETHING TO MAKE TOMORROW BETTER:

Day **14**

BREAKFAST

LUNCH

DINNER

SNACKS

EXERCISE / ACTIVITY

WATER

I SLEPT FOR

HOURS

CHALLENGES I FACED TODAY:

SOMETHING TO MAKE TOMORROW BETTER:

Day **15**

BREAKFAST LUNCH DINNER

SNACKS

EXERCISE / ACTIVITY

WATER

I SLEPT FOR

HOURS

CHALLENGES I FACED TODAY:

SOMETHING TO MAKE TOMORROW BETTER:

Day **16**

BREAKFAST   LUNCH   DINNER

SNACKS

EXERCISE / ACTIVITY

WATER

I SLEPT FOR

HOURS

CHALLENGES I FACED TODAY:

SOMETHING TO MAKE TOMORROW BETTER:

Day **17**

BREAKFAST	LUNCH	DINNER

SNACKS

EXERCISE / ACTIVITY

WATER

I SLEPT FOR

HOURS

CHALLENGES I FACED TODAY:

SOMETHING TO MAKE TOMORROW BETTER:

Day **18**

BREAKFAST	LUNCH	DINNER

SNACKS

EXERCISE / ACTIVITY

WATER

I SLEPT FOR

HOURS

CHALLENGES I FACED TODAY:

SOMETHING TO MAKE TOMORROW BETTER:

Day **19**

BREAKFAST   LUNCH   DINNER

SNACKS

EXERCISE / ACTIVITY

WATER

I SLEPT FOR

HOURS

CHALLENGES I FACED TODAY:

SOMETHING TO MAKE TOMORROW BETTER:

Day 20

BREAKFAST   LUNCH   DINNER

SNACKS

EXERCISE / ACTIVITY

WATER

I SLEPT FOR

HOURS

CHALLENGES I FACED TODAY:

SOMETHING TO MAKE TOMORROW BETTER:

Day **21**

BREAKFAST   LUNCH   DINNER

SNACKS

EXERCISE / ACTIVITY

WATER

I SLEPT FOR

HOURS

CHALLENGES I FACED TODAY:

SOMETHING TO MAKE TOMORROW BETTER:

Day 22

BREAKFAST

LUNCH

DINNER

SNACKS

EXERCISE / ACTIVITY

WATER

I SLEPT FOR

HOURS

CHALLENGES I FACED TODAY:

SOMETHING TO MAKE TOMORROW BETTER:

Day **23**

BREAKFAST	LUNCH	DINNER

SNACKS

EXERCISE / ACTIVITY

WATER

I SLEPT FOR

HOURS

CHALLENGES I FACED TODAY:

SOMETHING TO MAKE TOMORROW BETTER:

Day 24

BREAKFAST   LUNCH   DINNER

SNACKS

EXERCISE / ACTIVITY

WATER

I SLEPT FOR

HOURS

CHALLENGES I FACED TODAY:

SOMETHING TO MAKE TOMORROW BETTER:

Day **25**

BREAKFAST	LUNCH	DINNER

SNACKS

EXERCISE / ACTIVITY

WATER

I SLEPT FOR

HOURS

CHALLENGES I FACED TODAY:

SOMETHING TO MAKE TOMORROW BETTER:

Day **26**

BREAKFAST

LUNCH

DINNER

SNACKS

EXERCISE / ACTIVITY

WATER

I SLEPT FOR

HOURS

CHALLENGES I FACED TODAY:

SOMETHING TO MAKE TOMORROW BETTER:

Day **27**

BREAKFAST   LUNCH   DINNER

SNACKS

EXERCISE / ACTIVITY

WATER

I SLEPT FOR

HOURS

CHALLENGES I FACED TODAY:

SOMETHING TO MAKE TOMORROW BETTER:

Day 28

BREAKFAST

LUNCH

DINNER

SNACKS

EXERCISE / ACTIVITY

WATER

I SLEPT FOR

HOURS

CHALLENGES I FACED TODAY:

SOMETHING TO MAKE TOMORROW BETTER:

Day 29

BREAKFAST   LUNCH   DINNER

SNACKS

EXERCISE / ACTIVITY

WATER

I SLEPT FOR

HOURS

CHALLENGES I FACED TODAY:

SOMETHING TO MAKE TOMORROW BETTER:

Day **30**

BREAKFAST   LUNCH   DINNER

SNACKS

EXERCISE / ACTIVITY

WATER

I SLEPT FOR

HOURS

CHALLENGES I FACED TODAY:

SOMETHING TO MAKE TOMORROW BETTER:

Boom! You've formed new habits!

DAY 30

Congrats on completing your first 30 days! Hopefully you've written down everything you've eaten and noted any physical activity too. You're learning new habits every day. Now, grab the tape measure and see what your new body measurements are. Then squeal with delight because you're killing it!

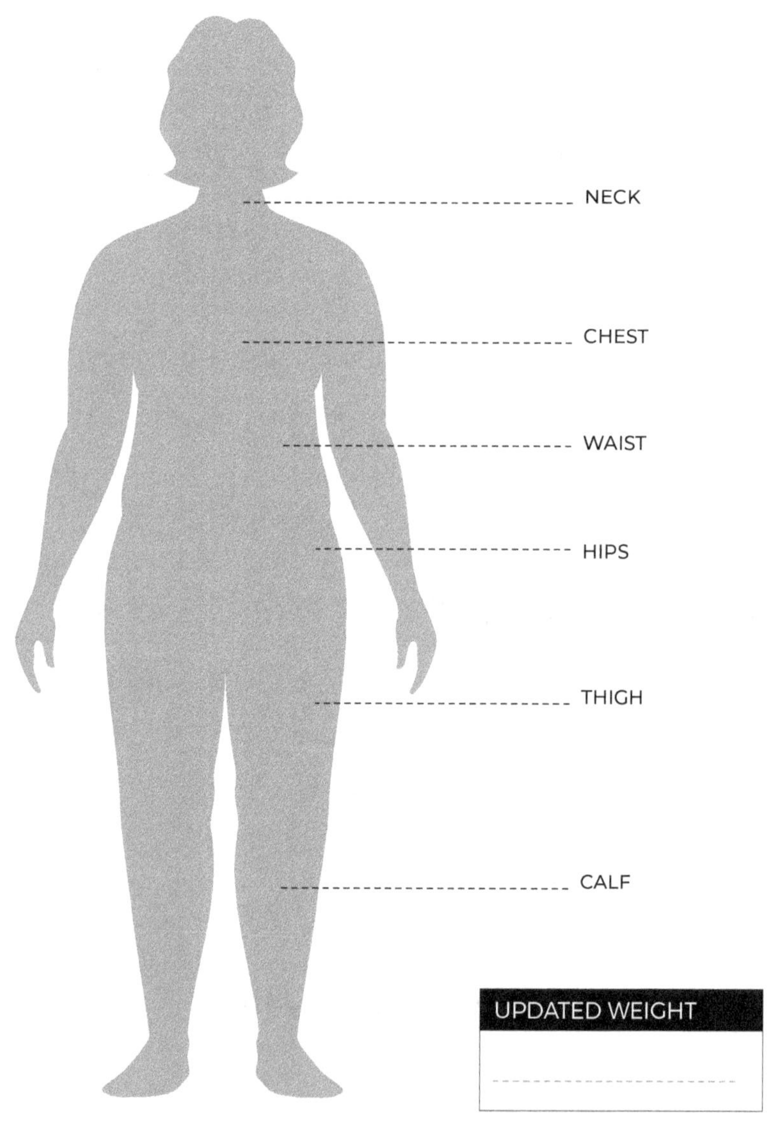

UPDATED WEIGHT

Day **31**

BREAKFAST   LUNCH   DINNER

SNACKS

EXERCISE / ACTIVITY

WATER

I SLEPT FOR

HOURS

CHALLENGES I FACED TODAY:

SOMETHING TO MAKE TOMORROW BETTER:

Day **32**

BREAKFAST	LUNCH	DINNER

SNACKS

EXERCISE / ACTIVITY

WATER

I SLEPT FOR

HOURS

CHALLENGES I FACED TODAY:

SOMETHING TO MAKE TOMORROW BETTER:

Day **33**

BREAKFAST	LUNCH	DINNER

SNACKS

EXERCISE / ACTIVITY

WATER

I SLEPT FOR

HOURS

CHALLENGES I FACED TODAY:

SOMETHING TO MAKE TOMORROW BETTER:

Day **34**

BREAKFAST　　　　　LUNCH　　　　　DINNER

SNACKS

EXERCISE / ACTIVITY

WATER

I SLEPT FOR

HOURS

CHALLENGES I FACED TODAY:

SOMETHING TO MAKE TOMORROW BETTER:

Day **35**

BREAKFAST   LUNCH   DINNER

SNACKS

EXERCISE / ACTIVITY

WATER

I SLEPT FOR

HOURS

CHALLENGES I FACED TODAY:

SOMETHING TO MAKE TOMORROW BETTER:

Day **36**

BREAKFAST   LUNCH   DINNER

SNACKS

EXERCISE / ACTIVITY

WATER

I SLEPT FOR

HOURS

CHALLENGES I FACED TODAY:

SOMETHING TO MAKE TOMORROW BETTER:

Day **37**

BREAKFAST

LUNCH

DINNER

SNACKS

EXERCISE / ACTIVITY

WATER

I SLEPT FOR

HOURS

CHALLENGES I FACED TODAY:

SOMETHING TO MAKE TOMORROW BETTER:

Day **38**

BREAKFAST	LUNCH	DINNER

SNACKS

EXERCISE / ACTIVITY

WATER

I SLEPT FOR

HOURS

CHALLENGES I FACED TODAY:

SOMETHING TO MAKE TOMORROW BETTER:

Day **39**

BREAKFAST LUNCH DINNER

SNACKS

EXERCISE / ACTIVITY

WATER

I SLEPT FOR

HOURS

CHALLENGES I FACED TODAY:

SOMETHING TO MAKE TOMORROW BETTER:

Day **40**

BREAKFAST   LUNCH   DINNER

SNACKS

EXERCISE / ACTIVITY

WATER

I SLEPT FOR

HOURS

CHALLENGES I FACED TODAY:

SOMETHING TO MAKE TOMORROW BETTER:

Day **41**

BREAKFAST

LUNCH

DINNER

SNACKS

EXERCISE / ACTIVITY

WATER

I SLEPT FOR

HOURS

CHALLENGES I FACED TODAY:

SOMETHING TO MAKE TOMORROW BETTER:

Day **42**

BREAKFAST	LUNCH	DINNER

SNACKS

EXERCISE / ACTIVITY

WATER

I SLEPT FOR

HOURS

CHALLENGES I FACED TODAY:

SOMETHING TO MAKE TOMORROW BETTER:

Day **43**

BREAKFAST   LUNCH   DINNER

SNACKS

EXERCISE / ACTIVITY

WATER

I SLEPT FOR

HOURS

CHALLENGES I FACED TODAY:

SOMETHING TO MAKE TOMORROW BETTER:

Day **44**

BREAKFAST   LUNCH   DINNER

SNACKS

EXERCISE / ACTIVITY

WATER

I SLEPT FOR

HOURS

CHALLENGES I FACED TODAY:

SOMETHING TO MAKE TOMORROW BETTER:

Day **45**

BREAKFAST

LUNCH

DINNER

SNACKS

EXERCISE / ACTIVITY

WATER

I SLEPT FOR

HOURS

CHALLENGES I FACED TODAY:

SOMETHING TO MAKE TOMORROW BETTER:

Day **46**

BREAKFAST   LUNCH   DINNER

SNACKS

EXERCISE / ACTIVITY

WATER

I SLEPT FOR

HOURS

CHALLENGES I FACED TODAY:

SOMETHING TO MAKE TOMORROW BETTER:

Day **47**

BREAKFAST   LUNCH   DINNER

SNACKS

EXERCISE / ACTIVITY

WATER

I SLEPT FOR

HOURS

CHALLENGES I FACED TODAY:

SOMETHING TO MAKE TOMORROW BETTER:

Day **48**

BREAKFAST   LUNCH   DINNER

SNACKS

EXERCISE / ACTIVITY

WATER

I SLEPT FOR

HOURS

CHALLENGES I FACED TODAY:

SOMETHING TO MAKE TOMORROW BETTER:

Day **49**

BREAKFAST

LUNCH

DINNER

SNACKS

EXERCISE / ACTIVITY

WATER

I SLEPT FOR

HOURS

CHALLENGES I FACED TODAY:

SOMETHING TO MAKE TOMORROW BETTER:

Day **50**

BREAKFAST   LUNCH   DINNER

SNACKS

EXERCISE / ACTIVITY

WATER

I SLEPT FOR

HOURS

CHALLENGES I FACED TODAY:

SOMETHING TO MAKE TOMORROW BETTER:

Day 51

BREAKFAST

LUNCH

DINNER

SNACKS

EXERCISE / ACTIVITY

WATER

I SLEPT FOR

HOURS

CHALLENGES I FACED TODAY:

SOMETHING TO MAKE TOMORROW BETTER:

Day **52**

BREAKFAST   LUNCH   DINNER

SNACKS

EXERCISE / ACTIVITY

WATER

I SLEPT FOR

HOURS

CHALLENGES I FACED TODAY:

SOMETHING TO MAKE TOMORROW BETTER:

Day **53**

BREAKFAST   LUNCH   DINNER

SNACKS

EXERCISE / ACTIVITY

WATER

I SLEPT FOR

HOURS

CHALLENGES I FACED TODAY:

SOMETHING TO MAKE TOMORROW BETTER:

Day **54**

BREAKFAST	LUNCH	DINNER

SNACKS

EXERCISE / ACTIVITY

WATER

I SLEPT FOR

HOURS

CHALLENGES I FACED TODAY:

SOMETHING TO MAKE TOMORROW BETTER:

Day **55**

BREAKFAST   **LUNCH**   **DINNER**

SNACKS

EXERCISE / ACTIVITY

WATER

I SLEPT FOR

HOURS

CHALLENGES I FACED TODAY:

SOMETHING TO MAKE TOMORROW BETTER:

Day **56**

BREAKFAST   LUNCH   DINNER

SNACKS

EXERCISE / ACTIVITY

WATER

I SLEPT FOR

HOURS

CHALLENGES I FACED TODAY:

SOMETHING TO MAKE TOMORROW BETTER:

Day **57**

BREAKFAST   LUNCH   DINNER

SNACKS

EXERCISE / ACTIVITY

WATER

I SLEPT FOR

HOURS

CHALLENGES I FACED TODAY:

SOMETHING TO MAKE TOMORROW BETTER:

Day **58**

BREAKFAST	LUNCH	DINNER

SNACKS

EXERCISE / ACTIVITY

WATER

I SLEPT FOR

HOURS

CHALLENGES I FACED TODAY:

SOMETHING TO MAKE TOMORROW BETTER:

Day **59**

BREAKFAST

LUNCH

DINNER

SNACKS

EXERCISE / ACTIVITY

WATER

I SLEPT FOR

HOURS

CHALLENGES I FACED TODAY:

SOMETHING TO MAKE TOMORROW BETTER:

Day **60**

BREAKFAST   LUNCH   DINNER

SNACKS

EXERCISE / ACTIVITY

WATER

I SLEPT FOR

HOURS

CHALLENGES I FACED TODAY:

SOMETHING TO MAKE TOMORROW BETTER:

You are a superstar!

DAY 60

Holy sh*t you're doing it! You're well over halfway now and should be seeing some real differences in your daily habits and health. Take a moment to remember WHY you're doing this and prepare to knock the next 30 days out of the park. Update your digits below and be in awe of your greatness!

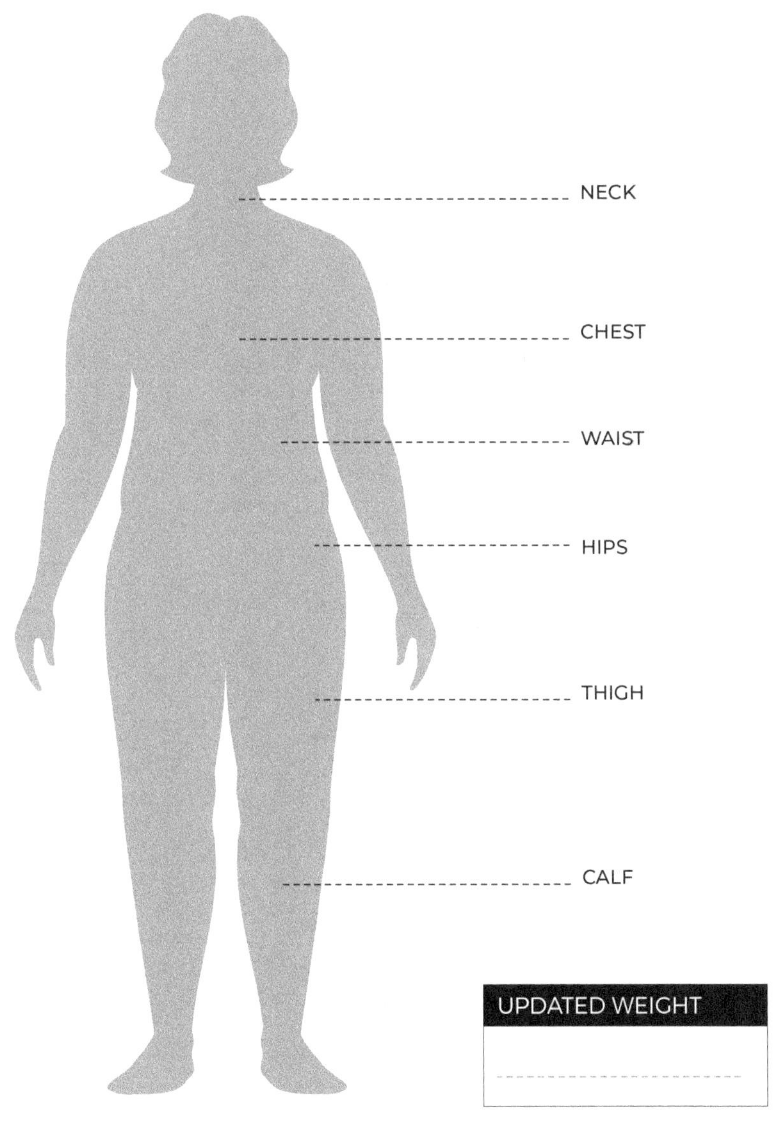

UPDATED WEIGHT

Day **61**

BREAKFAST   LUNCH   DINNER

SNACKS

EXERCISE / ACTIVITY

WATER

I SLEPT FOR

HOURS

CHALLENGES I FACED TODAY:

SOMETHING TO MAKE TOMORROW BETTER:

Day **62**

BREAKFAST	LUNCH	DINNER

SNACKS

EXERCISE / ACTIVITY

WATER

I SLEPT FOR

HOURS

CHALLENGES I FACED TODAY:

SOMETHING TO MAKE TOMORROW BETTER:

Day **63**

BREAKFAST	LUNCH	DINNER

SNACKS

EXERCISE / ACTIVITY

WATER

I SLEPT FOR

HOURS

CHALLENGES I FACED TODAY:

SOMETHING TO MAKE TOMORROW BETTER:

Day **64**

BREAKFAST   LUNCH   DINNER

SNACKS

EXERCISE / ACTIVITY

WATER

I SLEPT FOR

HOURS

CHALLENGES I FACED TODAY:

SOMETHING TO MAKE TOMORROW BETTER:

Day **65**

BREAKFAST   LUNCH   DINNER

SNACKS

EXERCISE / ACTIVITY

WATER

I SLEPT FOR

HOURS

CHALLENGES I FACED TODAY:

SOMETHING TO MAKE TOMORROW BETTER:

Day **66**

BREAKFAST   LUNCH   DINNER

SNACKS

EXERCISE / ACTIVITY

WATER

I SLEPT FOR

HOURS

CHALLENGES I FACED TODAY:

SOMETHING TO MAKE TOMORROW BETTER:

Day **67**

BREAKFAST	LUNCH	DINNER

SNACKS

EXERCISE / ACTIVITY

WATER

I SLEPT FOR

HOURS

CHALLENGES I FACED TODAY:

SOMETHING TO MAKE TOMORROW BETTER:

Day **68**

BREAKFAST	LUNCH	DINNER

SNACKS

EXERCISE / ACTIVITY

WATER

I SLEPT FOR

HOURS

CHALLENGES I FACED TODAY:

SOMETHING TO MAKE TOMORROW BETTER:

Day **69**

BREAKFAST   LUNCH   DINNER

SNACKS

EXERCISE / ACTIVITY

WATER

I SLEPT FOR

HOURS

CHALLENGES I FACED TODAY:

SOMETHING TO MAKE TOMORROW BETTER:

Day **70**

BREAKFAST   LUNCH   DINNER

SNACKS

EXERCISE / ACTIVITY

WATER

I SLEPT FOR

HOURS

CHALLENGES I FACED TODAY:

SOMETHING TO MAKE TOMORROW BETTER:

Day **71**

BREAKFAST   LUNCH   DINNER

SNACKS

EXERCISE / ACTIVITY

WATER

I SLEPT FOR

HOURS

CHALLENGES I FACED TODAY:

SOMETHING TO MAKE TOMORROW BETTER:

Day **72**

BREAKFAST   LUNCH   DINNER

SNACKS

EXERCISE / ACTIVITY

WATER

I SLEPT FOR

HOURS

CHALLENGES I FACED TODAY:

SOMETHING TO MAKE TOMORROW BETTER:

Day **73**

BREAKFAST	LUNCH	DINNER

SNACKS

EXERCISE / ACTIVITY

WATER

I SLEPT FOR

HOURS

CHALLENGES I FACED TODAY:

SOMETHING TO MAKE TOMORROW BETTER:

Day **74**

BREAKFAST   LUNCH   DINNER

SNACKS

EXERCISE / ACTIVITY

WATER

I SLEPT FOR

HOURS

CHALLENGES I FACED TODAY:

SOMETHING TO MAKE TOMORROW BETTER:

Day **75**

BREAKFAST	LUNCH	DINNER

SNACKS

EXERCISE / ACTIVITY

WATER

I SLEPT FOR

HOURS

CHALLENGES I FACED TODAY:

SOMETHING TO MAKE TOMORROW BETTER:

Day **76**

BREAKFAST   LUNCH   DINNER

SNACKS

EXERCISE / ACTIVITY

WATER

I SLEPT FOR

HOURS

CHALLENGES I FACED TODAY:

SOMETHING TO MAKE TOMORROW BETTER:

Day **77**

BREAKFAST   LUNCH   DINNER

SNACKS

EXERCISE / ACTIVITY

WATER

I SLEPT FOR

HOURS

CHALLENGES I FACED TODAY:

SOMETHING TO MAKE TOMORROW BETTER:

Day **78**

BREAKFAST

LUNCH

DINNER

SNACKS

EXERCISE / ACTIVITY

WATER

I SLEPT FOR

HOURS

CHALLENGES I FACED TODAY:

SOMETHING TO MAKE TOMORROW BETTER:

Day **79**

BREAKFAST	LUNCH	DINNER

SNACKS

EXERCISE / ACTIVITY

WATER

I SLEPT FOR

HOURS

CHALLENGES I FACED TODAY:

SOMETHING TO MAKE TOMORROW BETTER:

Day **80**

BREAKFAST LUNCH DINNER

SNACKS

EXERCISE / ACTIVITY

WATER

I SLEPT FOR

HOURS

CHALLENGES I FACED TODAY:

SOMETHING TO MAKE TOMORROW BETTER:

Day 81

BREAKFAST	LUNCH	DINNER

SNACKS

EXERCISE / ACTIVITY

WATER

I SLEPT FOR

HOURS

CHALLENGES I FACED TODAY:

SOMETHING TO MAKE TOMORROW BETTER:

Day **82**

BREAKFAST   LUNCH   DINNER

SNACKS

EXERCISE / ACTIVITY

WATER

I SLEPT FOR

HOURS

CHALLENGES I FACED TODAY:

SOMETHING TO MAKE TOMORROW BETTER:

Day **83**

BREAKFAST	LUNCH	DINNER

SNACKS

EXERCISE / ACTIVITY

WATER

I SLEPT FOR

HOURS

CHALLENGES I FACED TODAY:

SOMETHING TO MAKE TOMORROW BETTER:

Day 84

BREAKFAST

LUNCH

DINNER

SNACKS

EXERCISE / ACTIVITY

WATER

I SLEPT FOR

HOURS

CHALLENGES I FACED TODAY:

SOMETHING TO MAKE TOMORROW BETTER:

Day **85**

BREAKFAST	LUNCH	DINNER

SNACKS

EXERCISE / ACTIVITY

WATER

I SLEPT FOR

HOURS

CHALLENGES I FACED TODAY:

SOMETHING TO MAKE TOMORROW BETTER:

Day **86**

BREAKFAST   LUNCH   DINNER

SNACKS

EXERCISE / ACTIVITY

WATER

I SLEPT FOR

HOURS

CHALLENGES I FACED TODAY:

SOMETHING TO MAKE TOMORROW BETTER:

Day **87**

BREAKFAST   LUNCH   DINNER

SNACKS

EXERCISE / ACTIVITY

WATER

I SLEPT FOR

HOURS

CHALLENGES I FACED TODAY:

SOMETHING TO MAKE TOMORROW BETTER:

Day **88**

BREAKFAST

LUNCH

DINNER

SNACKS

EXERCISE / ACTIVITY

WATER

I SLEPT FOR

HOURS

CHALLENGES I FACED TODAY:

SOMETHING TO MAKE TOMORROW BETTER:

Day **89**

BREAKFAST
LUNCH
DINNER

SNACKS

EXERCISE / ACTIVITY

WATER

I SLEPT FOR

HOURS

CHALLENGES I FACED TODAY:

SOMETHING TO MAKE TOMORROW BETTER:

Day **90**

BREAKFAST	LUNCH	DINNER

SNACKS

EXERCISE / ACTIVITY

WATER

I SLEPT FOR

HOURS

CHALLENGES I FACED TODAY:

SOMETHING TO MAKE TOMORROW BETTER:

Congratulations!

DAY 90

Hello New You! You've done it! You've nailed new habits and written in this journal every day for the past 90 days! Bragging rights are yours once you've taken your last measurements below.

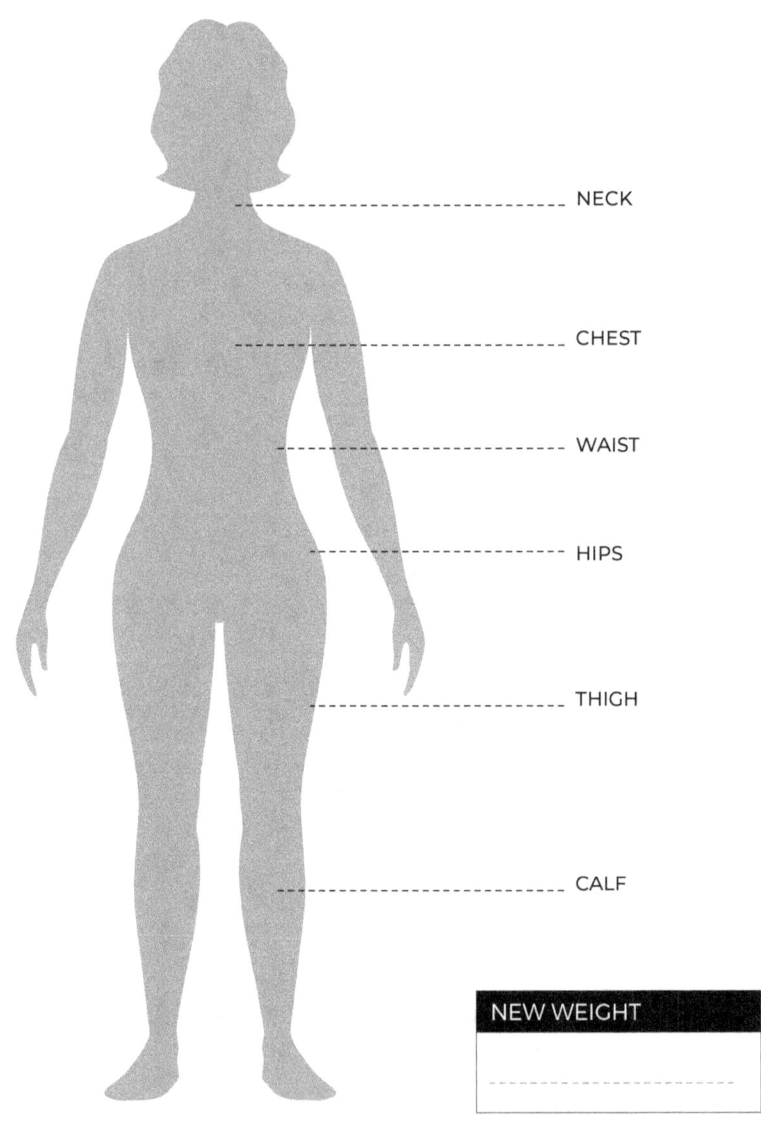

NEW WEIGHT

Be proud...

Take a moment now and reflect on what you've achieved.
You've learned new habits.
You've committed to making a better YOU.
You've sorted out your sh*t, and now you can be super proud of your
efforts. Tracking your daily food and fitness means you've become more
aware of what you're putting into your body, and the impact it has.

Keep those habits up and shine glorious one... **SHINE!**